**Disclaimer**

This book is intended to help people become better informed medical consumers. The information in this book is intended to supplement, not replace, the medical advice of a trained health care professional. No mention or description of uses of drugs listed herein should be construed as an endorsement of those uses or drugs. Only a physician can prescribe drugs and their precise dosages. All matters regarding your health require medical supervision. The authors and publisher disclaim any liability arising directly or indirectly from use of this book.

**Notice of rights**

All rights reserved for the book itself: this book may not be reproduced or transmitted in any form by any means, electronic, mechanical, photocopying, recording, or otherwise, without the prior written permission of the publisher.

The information in this book is distributed on an "As Is" basis without warranty. While every precaution has been taken in the preparation of he book, neither the author nor the publisher shall have any liability to any person or entity with respect to any loss or damage caused or alleged to be caused directly or indirectly by the instructions contained in this book or by the products described in it.

**Trademarks**

Many of the designations used by manufacturers and sellers to distinguish their products are claimed as trademarks. Where those designations appear in this book, and the publisher was aware of a trademark claim, the designations appear as requested by the owner of the trademark. All other product names and services identified throughout this book are used in editorial fashion only and for the benefit of such companies with no intention of infringement of the trademark. No such use, or the use of any trade name, is intended to convey endorsement or other affiliation with this book.

Copyright © by G.J. Blokdijk

# Table of Contents

| | |
|---|---|
| Your feedback is invaluable to us | 3 |
| Why use this book? | 3 |
| How to use this book? | 4 |
| BEGINNING OF THE QUESTION CHAPTERS: | 6 |
| CHAPTER #1: WHO: | 7 |
| CHAPTER #2: WHAT: | 22 |
| CHAPTER #3: WHERE: | 54 |
| CHAPTER #4: WHEN: | 69 |
| CHAPTER #5: WHY: | 84 |
| CHAPTER #6: HOW: | 98 |
| CHAPTER #7: HOW MUCH: | 114 |
| Index | 129 |

# Your feedback is invaluable to us

If you recently bought this book, we would love to hear from you! You can do this by writing a review on amazon (or the online store where you purchased this book) about your last purchase! As part of our continual service improvement process, we love to hear real client experiences and feedback.

**How does it work?**
To post a review on Amazon, just log in to your account and click on the Create Your Own Review button (under Customer Reviews) of the relevant product page. You can find examples of product reviews in Amazon. If you purchased from another online store, simply follow their procedures.

# Why use this book?

Everyone should ask questions when getting a prescription. This is especially important when your doctor or other health care professional prescribes you Pancuronium Bromide.

What should you ask?

Your health depends on good communication, but which questions to ask your doctor? Having the right questions is the answer.

Asking questions and providing information to your doctor and other care providers can improve your care. Talking with your doctor builds trust and leads to better satisfaction, quality, safety and results.

Asking questions is key to good communication with your doctor. If you do not ask questions, he or she may assume you already know the answer or that you do not want more information. Do not wait for the doctor to raise a specific question or subject; he or she may not know it is important to you. Be proactive. Ask questions.

Effective health care is a team effort. You are part of this team and play an important role. One of the best ways to communicate with your doctor and health care team is by asking questions. Since time is limited when you have your medical appointments, you will feel less rushed when you prepare your questions before your appointment.

Your doctor wants your questions. Doctors know a lot about a lot of things, but they do not always know everything about you, what you want to know or what is best for you.

Your questions give your doctor and health care professionals important information about you, like your most important health care concerns.

That is why they need you to speak up.

## How to use this book?

When you meet with your doctor or other members of your health care team, you will hear a lot of information. It helps to think ahead of time of the things you want to know and to highlight the questions in this book you want to ask and take this book with you to your appointments.

This book contains questions you may want to ask your doctor. You should use the questions that fit your situation, and skip those that do not apply.

This book offers many ways that you can ask questions and get your health care needs met. With this book you will have numerous simple questions that can help you take better care of yourself, feel better, and get the right care at the right time.

Doctors and medical professionals want to know your questions to help them take better care of you and offer advice to get your most pressing questions answered.

Be prepared for your next medical appointment. Take this book with you if you are getting a checkup, want to discuss a problem or health condition, are getting a prescription, or talk about a medical test or surgery and be sure to write down the answers your health care professional provides for you in this book.

Whatever the reason for your appointment, it is important to be prepared.

Take charge of your health. Ask your health care providers questions and learn about the Pancuronium Bromide medicine you take.

**BEGINNING OF THE QUESTION CHAPTERS:**

# CHAPTER #1: WHO:

INTENT: Who benefits from Pancuronium Bromide (Is this right for me.)

**1. Will I be able to do _____ after treatment?**

Notes:

2. Is this normal or should I see a shrink for Pancuronium Bromide medication?

Notes:

3. Can I share Pancuronium Bromide prescription drugs?

Notes:

4. How do you prevent re-admission in case I forget to take my Pancuronium Bromide prescription

medications. How do you help those who have problems following suggestions regarding eating habits, smoking, drinking, and taking drugs..?

Notes:

5. Who can join a Medicare Pancuronium Bromide prescription drug plan?

Notes:

6. Is it true that an online pharmacy can save me money on Pancuronium Bromide prescription drugs?

Notes:

**7. Do we have to do this now - or can we revisit it later?**

Notes:

8. Who typically uses Pancuronium Bromide prescription drugs, and where do they get them?

Notes:

**9. Will I be able to take my prescription medications after surgery?**

Notes:


10. Is sharing Pancuronium Bromide prescription drugs illegal?

Notes:


**11. Where can US citizens buy their prescription drugs online from legally, in confidence, and under which conditions?**

Notes:


**12. I Googled my symptoms and read this. Is it accurate?**

Notes:


13. Does it matter at what time I use my Pancuronium Bromide medication?

Notes:

14. They say _____ not to take this with Pancuronium Bromide prescription medication, but do you think it will hurt me?

Notes:

**15. What does using a prescription drug Off-label mean?**

Notes:

**16. Are there simpler - safer options?**

Notes:

17. Who can get Medicare Pancuronium Bromide prescription drug coverage?

Notes:

18. Who is eligible to receive Pancuronium Bromide prescription drug help?

Notes:

**19. Is there anything else I should be asking?**

Notes:

20. Who is qualified to receive Pancuronium Bromide prescription drug help?

Notes:

21. How can a wholesome mud-bath help my condition, and what is the effect on my Pancuronium Bromide prescription drugs?

Notes:

**22. What is the Prescription Drug Monitoring Database and who is using it?**

Notes:

23. Who can I contact if I want to meet with a specialist for long-term Pancuronium Bromide medication management on an ongoing basis?

Notes:

**24. Do generic medications have the exact same**

**ingredients?**

Notes:

25. Can Pancuronium Bromide medication cause hair loss?

Notes:

26. Can you help me save money on my Pancuronium Bromide prescription medication?

Notes:

27. Who should NOT take Pancuronium Bromide medication?

Notes:

28. What are generic alternatives for my Pancuronium Bromide prescription drugs?

Notes:

29. Can my baby get harmed by my Pancuronium Bromide prescription drug use?

Notes:



30. So who approves these Pancuronium Bromide medications?

Notes:



31. Can you help me with finding the money to purchase doctor visits and also Pancuronium Bromide prescriptions medication?

Notes:



32. Who is accountable for my Pancuronium Bromide prescription drug use?

Notes:



33. What exactly is this Pancuronium Bromide medication for in my case and how do you think it is working so well?

Notes:



34. How do I get my Pancuronium Bromide

medication without prescription drug coverage?

Notes:

35. Who gets to see the Pancuronium Bromide prescription drug information submitted in my patient medical questionnaire?

Notes:

36. Can enzymes be taken with other Pancuronium Bromide prescription medications?

Notes:

37. Will Pancuronium Bromide cause a mood change?

Notes:

38. How do you help someone who has a Pancuronium Bromide prescription drugs addiction?

Notes:

39. Who gets Pancuronium Bromide, and when?

Notes:


40. Who is at risk for Pancuronium Bromide prescription drug addiction?

Notes:


41. Will any supplements interact with my Pancuronium Bromide prescription drugs?

Notes:


42. Are there any drug interactions if Pancuronium Bromide is taken in combination with other medications?

Notes:


43. Will any tests be necessary while I am taking Pancuronium Bromide medication?

Notes:


**44. Are any medications I am taking likely to cause breast problems?**

Notes:

45. Are there any side effects associated with this Pancuronium Bromide medication that I should know about?

Notes:

46. Has there been any follow up of those who have stopped taking Pancuronium Bromide medication?

Notes:

47. What is this Pancuronium Bromide medication for, why am I taking it?

Notes:

**48. When in care who is responsible for the MAR (Medication Administration Records), who can put information on to it and make changes?**

Notes:

49. Does Pancuronium Bromide medication work?

Notes:

50. Who is most susceptible to Pancuronium Bromide prescription drug abuse?

Notes:

51. Will Pancuronium Bromide have an effect on nausea?

Notes:

52. Can I take Pancuronium Bromide with my other medications?

Notes:

53. How to take Pancuronium Bromide medication?

Notes:

54. Who is validating my Pancuronium Bromide prescription drugs to make sure I am taking the correct pills?

Notes:

**55. I'm taking prescription medication abroad, will this be covered if it is lost or I run out?**

Notes:


56. Can enzymes be taken when a person is on Pancuronium Bromide prescription medications?

Notes:


57. Who makes this Pancuronium Bromide medication?

Notes:


58. If I am unable to comply with the treatment regimen, who else can administer Pancuronium Bromide medication?

Notes:


59. Do Pancuronium Bromide prescription drugs create new mental problems?

Notes:

60. How do I safely discard Pancuronium Bromide prescription drugs without having to worry?

Notes:

61. Would using Pancuronium Bromide mean that I would need my other medications less?

Notes:

**62. Can natural be just as potent, if not more potent than over-the-counter drugs, creams and ointments?**

Notes:

63. Are nutritional supplements safe to take if I am taking Pancuronium Bromide prescription medications?

Notes:

64. Can I continue to take Pancuronium Bromide prescription drugs over 10, 20 and 30 years or more?

Notes:

65. Who can assist with Pancuronium Bromide medication reminders?

Notes:

**66. Should I review my Medicare prescription drug plan choice every year?**

Notes:

67. Are generics available for all Pancuronium Bromide prescription drugs?

Notes:

**68. Can this test diagnose a problem or will I need further testing?**

Notes:

69. Can I take this Pancuronium Bromide medicine if I am pregnant?

Notes:

# CHAPTER #2: WHAT:

INTENT: What do I need to know about Pancuronium Bromide (What will it do for me and what can I expect.)

1. What Pancuronium Bromide prescription drugs have serious side effects?

Notes:

2. What are the important warnings for females taking Pancuronium Bromide?

Notes:

3. What are the causes of Pancuronium Bromide prescription drug abuse?

Notes:

**4. What outcome should I expect?**

Notes:

**5. What does a Pancuronium Bromide medication error involve?**

Notes:

**6. What Pancuronium Bromide medication should I take?**

Notes:

**7. What should you, as my doctor, know before prescribing Pancuronium Bromide medication?**

Notes:

**8. What about my regular medications, any interference with Pancuronium Bromide?**

Notes:

9. What is are food or drinks you recommend not to be taken with Pancuronium Bromide prescription medications?

Notes:

**10. What are the different treatment options?**

Notes:

**11. What prescription medications or off the shelf medicinal products would cause ringing in the ears?**

Notes:

12. What should I do if I miss my regular dose of Pancuronium Bromide?

Notes:

**13. What are the benefits of having the test?**

Notes:

14. What are my options if I have difficulty paying for

Pancuronium Bromide prescription drugs?

Notes:


**15. What will a negative result mean?**

Notes:


16. What is a 25/50 percent Pancuronium Bromide prescription drug plan?

Notes:


**17. In what situation would I need to go for counseling if I'm receiving medication treatment?**

Notes:


18. What kind of medication will I have to take, Pancuronium Bromide or anything else?

Notes:


**19. What sources can I trust?**

Notes:

**20. What can parents and other adults do to help prevent prescription drug abuse among youth?**

Notes:


21. What is a generic Pancuronium Bromide medication?

Notes:


22. What about alcohol and its effect on Pancuronium Bromide prescription drugs?

Notes:


23. What is the nature of the Pancuronium Bromide medications prescribed?

Notes:


**24. What is the safest way to dispose of unwanted medications?**

Notes:

25. What do you recommend to do with Pancuronium Bromide medication adherence being difficult for me since my busy life pulls me in multiple directions - can you help me understand the ramifications of non-adherence?

Notes:

**26. What questions haven't I asked that I should have?**

Notes:

27. Can you help me understand how much of my Pancuronium Bromide prescription drugs, equipment and services will be covered by my insurance and what I will have to pay?

Notes:

28. What are the Pancuronium Bromide medications I can take?

Notes:

**29. What will this test tell us?**

Notes:

30. What is the effect of Pancuronium Bromide on drowsiness?

Notes:

31. What are the signs and symptoms related to Pancuronium Bromide addiction?

Notes:

32. What replacement medications can you suggest for Pancuronium Bromide?

Notes:

33. What sexual response side effects can I expect from these Pancuronium Bromide medications?

Notes:

**34. What is a prescription drug error and how often and why do these errors occur??**

Notes:

35. What about taking a new Pancuronium Bromide medication?

Notes:

36. What is the brand name for the drug Pancuronium Bromide?

Notes:

37. At what point would you recommend Pancuronium Bromide prescription drugs, alternative therapies, or surgery?

Notes:

**38. What other sources are available, who can I talk to about this?**

Notes:

**39. What else can I do to treat my condition?**

Notes:

40. What are your thoughts on hypnotherapy and Pancuronium Bromide?

Notes:

41. What about side effects of Pancuronium Bromide?

Notes:

42. What is Pancuronium Bromide prescription drug detox?

Notes:

**43. What can I do to prevent my condition from recurring or worsening?**

Notes:

44. For what reasons would I have to be off Pancuronium Bromide medication and for how long?

Notes:

**45. What types of vitamins and supplements should I be taking?**

Notes:

**46. What happens if I have to cut my Pancuronium Bromide pills in half to make them last longer or skip a day of medication because I can't afford to buy it as often as it's prescribed?**

Notes:

**47. What are my risks of accidentally taking an overdose of Pancuronium Bromide prescription drugs?**

Notes:

**48. What is the effect of Pancuronium Bromide on infertility?**

Notes:

**49. What can I do to help win the war on prescription drug abuse?**

Notes:

50. What is my Pancuronium Bromide prescription drug benefit?

Notes:

**51. What's next?**

Notes:

52. What are the dosages of the Pancuronium Bromide medication?

Notes:

53. What are good reasons to not take my Pancuronium Bromide prescription medication?

Notes:

**54. What will a positive result mean?**

Notes:

**55. What causes my condition?**

Notes:


**56. What about my current medications or allergies and the effect on it of Pancuronium Bromide?**

Notes:


**57. What lifestyle changes can change my condition?**

Notes:


**58. What is the proper course of treatment for me?**

Notes:


59. What other prescription drugs should I avoid while taking my Pancuronium Bromide medicines?

Notes:


60. What is a generic Pancuronium Bromide medication or drug, what does that term mean and what can it do for me?

Notes:

61. Is Pancuronium Bromide safe when breastfeeding, what are the effects on nursing?

Notes:

62. Besides Pancuronium Bromide medication, what else to do?

Notes:

63. What are your experiences with Pancuronium Bromide prescription drugs?

Notes:

**64. What medications have you yourself used in the past to make yourself better?**

Notes:

65. What kind of Pancuronium Bromide medications do the varying plans offer and how much can I save?

Notes:

66. What's the difference between all of the Pancuronium Bromide's class medications?

Notes:

**67. What else could I be doing to stay healthy and prevent disease?**

Notes:

68. What if my prescription Pancuronium Bromide medication is lost or stolen?

Notes:

**69. What medications are available to treat my condition?**

Notes:

70. What's the best mix for me of home remedies, over the counter (OTC) drugs and ointments and Pancuronium Bromide prescription drugs?

Notes:

71. Is it possible that my employer may look at what Pancuronium Bromide prescription medications I'm taking?

Notes:

72. What if I take Pancuronium Bromide prescription drugs and get little or no relief?

Notes:

73. What's to lose by trying another Pancuronium Bromide class medication?

Notes:

**74. What kind of resources do I have available to me?**

Notes:

75. What does this sign on my Pancuronium Bromide prescription drug imply?

Notes:

76. What is the name of my Pancuronium Bromide medication?

Notes:

**77. What if I'm taking other medication?**

Notes:

78. What happens if I stop using Pancuronium Bromide cold-turkey?

Notes:

79. What are the important warnings for males taking Pancuronium Bromide?

Notes:

80. What can I do to remember to take my Pancuronium Bromide medication?

Notes:

81. What if I have an allergic reaction to Pancuronium Bromide?

Notes:

**82. What is the evidence for this treatment?**

Notes:

83. What could be a natural alternative to more over-the-counter and Pancuronium Bromide prescription drugs?

Notes:

**84. What are some of the best non prescription medications I can give a try?**

Notes:

**85. What would you do if you were me?**

Notes:

86. Apart from Pancuronium Bromide medication, what are other components of your management plan?

Notes:


87. What are the Pancuronium Bromide medication side-effects?

Notes:


**88. What is my outcome?**

Notes:


89. What will happen to me without Pancuronium Bromide prescription drugs, diet, exercise, or nutritional supplements?

Notes:


**90. What kind of expectations should I have?**

Notes:


91. What if I'm already on medication and have side-

effects from the Pancuronium Bromide?

Notes:

92. What to eat, or what to use as a medication together with Pancuronium Bromide?

Notes:

**93. What is the branded prescription drug fee?**

Notes:

94. What can I expect from Pancuronium Bromide medication?

Notes:

95. What are the adverse health effects from Pancuronium Bromide prescription drugs?

Notes:

96. What if I am unhappy with the results of Pancuronium Bromide medication?

Notes:

**97. What's your go-to question for your own doctor?**

Notes:

98. What Pancuronium Bromide medications are used?

Notes:

**99. What should I do if I have other prescription drug coverage and want to join Medicare First?**

Notes:

**100. What are other treatment options?**

Notes:

**101. What happens if I don't do anything?**

Notes:

102. What would happen if I don't take the Pancuronium Bromide, would my health get worse?

Notes:

103. What's the probability that my Pancuronium Bromide medication is causing my symptoms?

Notes:

104. What will my Pancuronium Bromide medication do for me?

Notes:

105. What will be the net effect of Pancuronium Bromide medications for me?

Notes:

106. What is Pancuronium Bromide medication for?

Notes:

107. What should I expect after a procedure in terms

of soreness, what to watch for, Pancuronium Bromide medication, bathing, and level of activity?

Notes:

**108. What is the name of my condition, are there any other names it's known by?**

Notes:

109. What are my options in relation to Pancuronium Bromide medication, surgical procedures or remedy?

Notes:

**110. What medications should I ask for?**

Notes:

111. What if Pancuronium Bromide medication makes me gain weight?

Notes:

112. What if I am taking vitamins or over-the-counter drugs that could affect my Pancuronium Bromide

prescription drugs?

Notes:

113. What sort of Pancuronium Bromide prescription drug benefit is included?

Notes:

114. What are the side effects of the Pancuronium Bromide medication?

Notes:

115. How do scientists determine whether the chemical compounds in Pancuronium Bromide prescription medications do what they're claimed to do?

Notes:

**116. What is the prescription drug of choice for breakthrough pain meds?**

Notes:

117. What is the way to get my life back on track, without the unwanted side effects of Pancuronium Bromide prescription drugs?

Notes:

118. What exactly leads one to get dependent on Pancuronium Bromide prescription drugs?

Notes:

119. Will I need medication and what will it be, Pancuronium Bromide and/or anything else?

Notes:

120. What does my Pancuronium Bromide medication look like?

Notes:

121. What are my Pancuronium Bromide medication options?

Notes:

**122. Is treatment required, if so - what is it?**

Notes:


123. Do I need to change what I eat or stop any Pancuronium Bromide medications before doing a test?

Notes:


**124. What prescription drugs are you yourself taking?**

Notes:


125. What non-Pancuronium Bromide medications or vitamins should I take to speed up my healing?

Notes:


126. What really works as well as these Pancuronium Bromide medications, are there alternatives?

Notes:


127. What happens with my prescriptions for

Pancuronium Bromide medications while I am travelling overseas, how to get and fulfil those?

Notes:

128. What is the best approach if I forget to take this Pancuronium Bromide medication?

Notes:

129. What about Pancuronium Bromide's interactions with my medications?

Notes:

## 130. What if I am currently taking some other prescription medications?

Notes:

131. What other Pancuronium Bromide-like medications are in this class?

Notes:

## 132. What kind of experience with these issues do

**you have?**

Notes:

133. What types of Pancuronium Bromide medications are available?

Notes:

**134. How will you know what medications I am on?**

Notes:

135. What Pancuronium Bromide-like medications are safe to take during pregnancy?

Notes:

136. How will I benefit from working out in relation to my use of Pancuronium Bromide prescription medication, and what type of exercise would you recommend?

Notes:

**137. What will happen if I don't have the**

**treatment?**

Notes:


**138. What do I need to know about making the most of this Pancuronium Bromide prescription?**

Notes:


**139. What are the side effects?**

Notes:


**140. How do I book in to have the test and what is the usual waiting period?**

Notes:


**141. What if Pancuronium Bromide medication has changed since the application form was sent in?**

Notes:


**142. What if I have been taking Pancuronium Bromide medication with little to no relief?**

Notes:

143. What is the safest way to dispose of unused prescription Pancuronium Bromide medication?

Notes:

144. What is the easiest way to obtain the latest information about Pancuronium Bromide prescription drugs?

Notes:

145. What should I do if I experience side effects from the Pancuronium Bromide?

Notes:

146. What about Pancuronium Bromide prescription drug coverage?

Notes:

147. What should I know about Pancuronium Bromide medication?

Notes:

148. What medications can Pancuronium Bromide interact with?

Notes:

**149. In what way can mindfulness or meditation be useful?**

Notes:

150. What other drugs could interact with Pancuronium Bromide medication?

Notes:

151. What side effects can Pancuronium Bromide medication cause?

Notes:

**152. I want to read more about my condition. What online sources should I trust?**

Notes:

**153. What is the test for?**

Notes:



154. What Pancuronium Bromide's class medication can I take best?

Notes:



155. What if the Pancuronium Bromide medications produce unwelcome or harmful effects?

Notes:



156. What if I have tried various home remedies, over-the-counter medications or even Pancuronium Bromide prescription medications with no help?

Notes:



157. What medications on the market, OTC or Pancuronium Bromide prescription, can become harmful over time and would be dangerous if used well past the expiration date?

Notes:

# CHAPTER #3: WHERE:

INTENT: Where to next (Where can I find more information. Do i need a second opionion. What happens with tests.)

1. Does my plan cover my Pancuronium Bromide prescription drugs?

Notes:

**2. Where can I get more info about that?**

Notes:

3. What if my current Pancuronium Bromide prescription drugs are not on the formulary or are limited on the formulary?

Notes:

4. Will taking Pancuronium Bromide make me irritable?

Notes:


5. Where are others buying their Pancuronium Bromide prescription medications?

Notes:


**6. Are extended-release (ER) opioid medications optimum pain medications?**

Notes:


7. Will grapefruit affect my Pancuronium Bromide medications?

Notes:


8. If remedies help, what is the nature of Pancuronium Bromide medications and where could one go to explore them?

Notes:

**9. Will it help when I tell you about all my current medications and vitamin and herbal supplements?**

Notes:


10. Where else can I go for Pancuronium Bromide prescription medication, what are my options?

Notes:


11. What if I refuse the prescribed Pancuronium Bromide medication?

Notes:


12. May my employer ask me which Pancuronium Bromide prescription medications I am taking?

Notes:


**13. What if I take pain medication for _____?**

Notes:

14. Should I be on Pancuronium Bromide medication?

Notes:

15. Where are Pancuronium Bromide prescription drug users getting their prescription filled locally?

Notes:

16. Are side effects from Pancuronium Bromide medications the same in males and females?

Notes:

17. Is _____ a side effect of Pancuronium Bromide medication and is it permanent?

Notes:

18. Are there any other restrictions on Pancuronium Bromide prescription drug coverage?

Notes:

19. Is it possible to start with a solution which is natural and effective and less expensive than

Pancuronium Bromide prescription medication?

Notes:

20. Should I stop my Pancuronium Bromide medications before any procedure?

Notes:

21. Is there a Pancuronium Bromide prescription drug guide on the internet?

Notes:

22. Should I buy generic Pancuronium Bromide prescription medications?

Notes:

23. Does switching Pancuronium Bromide prescription drugs to over the counter as I age have any negative side effects?

Notes:

**24. Do you know of any medications available out**

**there that would help me be more comfortable?**

Notes:

25. How can I legally purchase Pancuronium Bromide prescription medications from Canada?

Notes:

26. Where do I go if I've run out of money and desperately need Pancuronium Bromide medication or a medical procedure?

Notes:

27. When you prescribe Pancuronium Bromide prescription medication for my condition, how do you weigh the side effects?

Notes:

28. What happens if I am willing to try new medications if the current Pancuronium Bromide ones are not working?

Notes:

29. Are these Pancuronium Bromide medications really helping?

Notes:



30. Where I can get a Pancuronium Bromide prescription drug?

Notes:



31. Should I be concerned about all the Pancuronium Bromide medication I need to take to stay on top of my health problems?

Notes:



32. If I do therapy, can I change or stop my Pancuronium Bromide medications?

Notes:



**33. Will I be able to carry enough prescription medications to avoid any health emergencies?**

Notes:

34. Could Pancuronium Bromide prescription medications cause a false positive on a test?

Notes:

35. Is Pancuronium Bromide a medicine with real evidence?

Notes:

**36. Will I have to take my medications forever?**

Notes:

**37. Can assisted living patients receive 90-day supplies of medications?**

Notes:

**38. What medications are safe for me to take during my pregnancy?**

Notes:

39. Should I take Pancuronium Bromide with other

medications?

Notes:


40. Are there any side effects of taking Pancuronium Bromide?

Notes:


41. Will you try and keep my Pancuronium Bromide medications at a level where I can function?

Notes:


42. Should I eat while taking specialized Pancuronium Bromide prescription drugs?

Notes:


43. Is Pancuronium Bromide safe if taking medications for high blood pressure?

Notes:


**44. How do I avoid getting in a place where I need so many prescription drugs to function?**

Notes:

### 45. Can I take the generic version of your prescription drugs?

Notes:

### 46. Which medication for my condition is right for me?

Notes:

47. What do each of these Pancuronium Bromide prescription medications have in common?

Notes:

### 48. How can you help me when I suffer from chronic pain, but am leery about taking prescription medication to help it?

Notes:

### 49. Should I get a second opinion?

Notes:

50. Where can I find info about taking more than one prescription medications together with Pancuronium Bromide?

Notes:

51. What are the effects of Pancuronium Bromide medications on cognition?

Notes:

52. How can I get Pancuronium Bromide prescription drug coverage?

Notes:

**53. May an employer ask all employees what prescription medications they are taking?**

Notes:

54. Will I get possible side neuritis of Pancuronium Bromide medications?

Notes:


**55. Is switching from one biologic medication to another effective?**

Notes:


**56. I take daily prescription medications, may I take my pills before I have my blood drawn?**

Notes:


57. Are the brands of Pancuronium Bromide prescription drugs I take covered?

Notes:


58. Please explain, what are the differences between generic and brand Pancuronium Bromide medications?

Notes:


**59. What are the best ways that do not require prescription medications to fall asleep faster?**

Notes:

**60. Did you wash your hands?**

Notes:

**61. Are there generic equivalents available for my Pancuronium Bromide prescription drugs?**

Notes:

**62. How do you handle potential prescription drug addiction and flow-on depression?**

Notes:

**63. Where would you send your partner or children?**

Notes:

**64. Can the Pancuronium Bromide medication cause substance abuse?**

Notes:

65. Where can I get my Pancuronium Bromide prescription medications filled?

Notes:

66. Where should I get my Pancuronium Bromide prescription drugs?

Notes:

67. Should I rely on Pancuronium Bromide, natural cures or over the counter medication?

Notes:

68. Where would I store my Pancuronium Bromide medications?

Notes:

**69. What if I start depending on antidepressants, alcohol, or other medications to calm me down or help me sleep?**

Notes:

# CHAPTER #4: WHEN:

> INTENT: When should I take or stop taking Pancuronium Bromide and how (When should I take it, stop taking it and how.)

1. Is it either / or when it comes to natural medicines and Pancuronium Bromide prescription drugs?

Notes:

2. Should I stop taking that Pancuronium Bromide medication?

Notes:

3. Have you instructed patients to discontinue taking their Pancuronium Bromide, or other prescription drugs?

Notes:

**4. Can I still take my current medications?**

Notes:

5. If I am stranded abroad and run out of my normal Pancuronium Bromide prescription medication, am I covered for this?

Notes:

6. Is there a certain Pancuronium Bromide or other medication that can improve my symptoms?

Notes:

7. Can all doctors prescribe Pancuronium Bromide Prescription Medication?

Notes:

8. When might herbal and nutritional therapies be a good alternative to over-the-counter and Pancuronium Bromide prescription medications for people with my condition?

Notes:

9. Do I need any Pancuronium Bromide medications?

Notes:

10. When does Pancuronium Bromide medication begin working?

Notes:

11. Can my child have his or her Pancuronium Bromide medication administered during the school day?

Notes:

12. Do you know all of the risks Pancuronium Bromide prescription drugs might pose?

Notes:

**13. Is there anything I should do to help prevent my health issue?**

Notes:

14. Do I need to take Pancuronium Bromide medications?

Notes:

**15. When and how will I get the results?**

Notes:

16. Is Pancuronium Bromide addictive?

Notes:

17. Do I have to be on more medications because of the side effects of Pancuronium Bromide?

Notes:

18. What are the Pancuronium Bromide prescription drug prices?

Notes:

19. Do vitamins interact with Pancuronium Bromide medications?

Notes:


20. Are you considering a trial of Pancuronium Bromide medications and/or anything else?

Notes:


21. What does one do when the only real help, the only Pancuronium Bromide medication available, no longer works?

Notes:


22. Is there financial help for Pancuronium Bromide prescription drugs?

Notes:


23. Can I take Pancuronium Bromide with other medications?

Notes:

24. When can seniors join a Pancuronium Bromide prescription drug plan?

Notes:


25. Are there safe Pancuronium Bromide-class prescription drugs available?

Notes:


**26. Do I really need this test?**

Notes:


27. Could a lot of the symptoms and brain fog I get be from the Pancuronium Bromide medications themselves?

Notes:


28. When I have been on the same amount of Pancuronium Bromide medication for years – when should that be re-evaluated?

Notes:

29. If acupuncture improves my condition, can I stop taking Pancuronium Bromide prescription medications?

Notes:


30. Can nutritional yeasts, especially brewers yeast, interact with Pancuronium Bromide medications?

Notes:


31. When should I be on Pancuronium Bromide medication?

Notes:


**32. What medications do I need to stop and when?**

Notes:


**33. How/when do I get test results?**

Notes:


34. Is it safe getting pregnant while on Pancuronium

Bromide medications?

Notes:


35. Could natural products be just as effective as Pancuronium Bromide prescription medications?

Notes:


**36. When will I know that I am taking excessive pain medication?**

Notes:


37. Are my Pancuronium Bromide medications safe to use while breastfeeding?

Notes:


38. What are some great ways to help remind me when to take Pancuronium Bromide medications?

Notes:


**39. What should I consider when buying coverage that provides prescription drug benefits?**

Notes:

**40. When did you graduate from medical school?**

Notes:

**41. Will these Pancuronium Bromide medications cause weight gain?**

Notes:

**42. Which of my medications cause the most weight gain?**

Notes:

**43. Are there any known Pancuronium Bromide prescription medication and chia seeds side effects when they are combined?**

Notes:

**44. Where can I buy Pancuronium Bromide prescription drugs cheaper?**

Notes:

45. Is there a generic version of the Pancuronium Bromide medication?

Notes:

46. Does Pancuronium Bromide medication and therapy work together?

Notes:

47. When should I stop using Pancuronium Bromide medication because of....?

Notes:

48. When should I take this Pancuronium Bromide medicine?

Notes:

**49. Do I need medication or surgery?**

Notes:

50. When could Pancuronium Bromide medication not be working anymore?

Notes:


**51. Should I have a current emergency contact form and a list of health conditions and medications readily available?**

Notes:


**52. Is it likely to get worse, or is it likely to get better?**

Notes:


53. Will I need any Pancuronium Bromide medication after surgery?

Notes:


54. Is it safe and legal to buy Pancuronium Bromide prescription drugs and other medications abroad?

Notes:

55. Can Reiki be used when taking Pancuronium Bromide medications?

Notes:

56. Is it okay to take my Pancuronium Bromide prescription drugs and multivitamin during a fast?

Notes:

57. If you have a Pancuronium Bromide prescription drug in your pocket, outside of the container when arrested is that considered DUI?

Notes:

58. How do I deal with any Pancuronium Bromide prescription medication when a side effect may be stated as 'may cause nausea or vomiting'?

Notes:

59. Should I bring my Pancuronium Bromide medications with me everywhere I go?

Notes:

**60. I feel like I need more medication, will you as my doctor be able to support me with my requests?**

Notes:


**61. Are there any risks involved in having this test?**

Notes:


62. How and when should I take my Pancuronium Bromide medication?

Notes:


63. What herbs, supplements, foods, drinks or activities should I avoid while taking Pancuronium Bromide medication?

Notes:


64. Can I safely use natural remedies and Pancuronium Bromide prescription drugs together?

Notes:

65. When should I stop taking Pancuronium Bromide medication?

Notes:

66. How will I know when my Pancuronium Bromide medications are working?

Notes:

67. When is it appropriate and safe to prescribe Pancuronium Bromide medication for my condition?

Notes:

68. When does this Pancuronium Bromide medication expire?

Notes:

**69. What are the differences between generic and brand medications?**

Notes:

# CHAPTER #5: WHY:

INTENT: Why do I need Pancuronium Bromide (Are there Alternatives. Why do I need it. Which symptoms does it medicate.)

1. Why is Pancuronium Bromide a prescription drug?

Notes:

2. Why is this Pancuronium Bromide medication prescribed?

Notes:

3. Should I really use this Pancuronium Bromide medication?

Notes:

4. Why do I need Pancuronium Bromide medicine?

Notes:

5. Why go the Pancuronium Bromide medication route?

Notes:

**6. Why are you doing this test?**

Notes:

**7. What does 50 deductible for brand name prescription drugs mean?**

Notes:

**8. Why have my bowel habits/appetite/mood/sex drive/etc changed?**

Notes:

**9. Are there any alternative tests?**

Notes:

**10. Why does my family's medical history matter, and what should I do about it?**

Notes:

11. How long will I need to take this Pancuronium Bromide medication?

Notes:

12. Which Pancuronium Bromide-like medication gives the most rapid relief?

Notes:

13. What should you do if I've messed up with my Pancuronium Bromide medication?

Notes:

**14. Um - can you explain that again?**

Notes:

15. Is Pancuronium Bromide medication the only answer for me?

Notes:


16. Are there any co-pays for medical treatments, hospitalization or Pancuronium Bromide prescription drugs?

Notes:


17. Do you offer treatment programs for those suffering from Pancuronium Bromide prescription drug addiction?

Notes:


18. Is Pancuronium Bromide as effective as other prescription medications?

Notes:


19. Why are Pancuronium Bromide medications so popular?

Notes:

20. If I am taking Pancuronium Bromide prescription medications can I take natural remedies?

Notes:

21. Who monitors the safety and effectiveness of Pancuronium Bromide prescription drugs?

Notes:

22. Why would I need Pancuronium Bromide prescription medication reminders?

Notes:

23. What would happen if I were suddenly unable to get access to my Pancuronium Bromide prescription drugs?

Notes:

24. Are Pancuronium Bromide medications safe for young kids?

Notes:

**25. Why are you giving me a blood test - and what will the results tell us?**

Notes:

**26. Are you aware of my personal medical history including current medications, allergies, and other considerations or limitations?**

Notes:

27. Do you have research you can share on Pancuronium Bromide prescription drug prices?

Notes:

28. Will Pancuronium Bromide cause me to test positive for various substances in a urine drug test?

Notes:

29. If I want to talk to a specialist in Pancuronium Bromide prescription drugs, where do I go?

Notes:


30. Are there any supplements or Pancuronium Bromide medications?

Notes:


**31. Is there an alternative medication?**

Notes:


**32. Why would I, while regularly taking prescription medications, have to approach grapefruit consumption with caution?**

Notes:


33. Could I have afforded it without Pancuronium Bromide prescription drug insurance?

Notes:


**34. How does my child at an out-of-state school obtain prescription drugs?**

Notes:

35. Will St. John's Wort interfere with Pancuronium Bromide prescription medications?

Notes:


36. Why is Pancuronium Bromide medication prescribed?

Notes:


37. Will you try and reach the primary reason for my problem before prescribing Pancuronium Bromide medications to solve my particular signs and symptoms?

Notes:


**38. Why and when use acupuncture for treating pain instead of, or combined with, taking pain medication?**

Notes:


39. Why is it important to take my Pancuronium Bromide prescription medication exactly as

prescribed?

Notes:



40. Precisely what are some good reasons Pancuronium Bromide prescription drugs can be recommended?

Notes:



**41. Is it all right for me to take allergy medication?**

Notes:



42. Will my Pancuronium Bromide prescription drugs build up toxins in my body?

Notes:



43. Can I take Pancuronium Bromide with prescription medication or with an underlying medical condition?

Notes:



44. Can we really know what is in Pancuronium Bromide prescription drugs?

Notes:

**45. Is there anything I can do on my own to improve my condition?**

Notes:

46. Is this worth getting Pancuronium Bromide medication for?

Notes:

47. If I take a Pancuronium Bromide medication, will it require more medication to counter the side effects?

Notes:

**48. Why are we doing these tests?**

Notes:

**49. What if I am currently without prescription drug coverage?**

Notes:

50. Which one of Pancuronium Bromide medications is better for me than the others?

Notes:

51. Will Pancuronium Bromide medication be the proper strength?

Notes:

**52. Can I use this app I found?**

Notes:

53. Will Pancuronium Bromide meet my expectations?

Notes:

54. Why do I need to manage Pancuronium Bromide medications?

Notes:

55. Can I expect any side effects from my Pancuronium Bromide medication?

Notes:

56. When is it time to think about why I'm on these Pancuronium Bromide drugs?

Notes:

57. Is there a non-prescription Pancuronium Bromide medication you might recommend?

Notes:

58. Do you have Pancuronium Bromide prescription drugs I can take throughout the day?

Notes:

59. Why is buying Pancuronium Bromide prescription drugs without a prescription dangerous?

Notes:

**60. Could you write it down?**

Notes:

**61. Why can't I buy some prescription drugs online?**

Notes:

62. Do individual policies pay for prescription Pancuronium Bromide medications?

Notes:

63. Can I take Pancuronium Bromide with my current medications?

Notes:

**64. Why does a prescription drug require authorization by a qualified professional and others do not?**

Notes:

65. Should I be worried about getting the wrong interaction if I combine Pancuronium Bromide

prescription drugs with natural supplements?

Notes:

66. Which Pancuronium Bromide-related prescription drugs are most dangerous?

Notes:

**67. Can I travel to _____ with prescription drugs used as medication for my condition?**

Notes:

68. Are all Pancuronium Bromide prescription drugs covered under health care plans?

Notes:

**69. If I have been taking the same prescription drugs for a long time, when is it time to evaluate?**

Notes:

# CHAPTER #6: HOW:

INTENT: How will Pancuronium Bromide affect me (How will it affect me negatively. How do I know if its a problem for me.)

1. How can Pancuronium Bromide medication be detected?

Notes:

**2. How long is it likely to last?**

Notes:

3. Is it probable to find out how to deal with my condition without taking Pancuronium Bromide prescription drugs?

Notes:

4. How should I use this Pancuronium Bromide medication?

Notes:


5. **How long will I need the treatment for?**

Notes:


6. How should this Pancuronium Bromide medication be taken?

Notes:


7. How do different Pancuronium Bromide-class prescription medications work differently?

Notes:


8. **How can I learn more about my symptoms or condition?**

Notes:

**9. How long will it take to get the results?**

Notes:


10. How are Pancuronium Bromide prescription drugs abused?

Notes:


11. How can I reduce my Pancuronium Bromide prescription drug costs?

Notes:


12. How to store Pancuronium Bromide medication?

Notes:


**13. How many surgeries do you perform each year?**

Notes:


14. So how do you know if you, or someone you love is having problems with Pancuronium Bromide

prescription drug abuse?

Notes:

15. How does Pancuronium Bromide prescription drug abuse start?

Notes:

16. How do I get better without Pancuronium Bromide medication?

Notes:

17. So I got a condition and a Pancuronium Bromide medication – how am I, as a patient, supposed to manage treatment?

Notes:

18. How do we order or pick up Pancuronium Bromide medications?

Notes:

19. My Pancuronium Bromide medications, just how

safe are they?

Notes:

20. How will I feel when I'm on Pancuronium Bromide medications?

Notes:

**21. How do generic medications compare in quality to brand name drugs?**

Notes:

22. How can I dispose of my Pancuronium Bromide prescription drugs safely?

Notes:

23. How will I know if the Pancuronium Bromide prescription and over-the-counter medications I take are interacting properly?

Notes:

24. How do I manage my Pancuronium Bromide

medications?

Notes:

25. How do I dispose of Pancuronium Bromide prescription medications?

Notes:

26. How will I know if my current Pancuronium Bromide Prescription Drug coverage is as good as the new Medicare Pancuronium Bromide Prescription Drug coverage?

Notes:

**27. How serious is this condition?**

Notes:

28. How about a new Pancuronium Bromide-like prescription drug?

Notes:

29. How wide-ranging is the Pancuronium Bromide

prescription drug coverage?

Notes:

30. How often is the Pancuronium Bromide medication taken?

Notes:

**31. How can I reduce or stop some of my medications?**

Notes:

32. Do you know how long it will take me to get my Pancuronium Bromide medication?

Notes:

**33. How often do I need to have the test done?**

Notes:

34. How long does the Pancuronium Bromide medication last?

Notes:

**35. Are there drugs to lift my mood, and how can this be achieved without prescription medications?**

Notes:

36. How can I make sure I am sufficiently stocked with the Pancuronium Bromide prescription medications I need?

Notes:

37. How can I find a few methods that can help my condition without the use of Pancuronium Bromide prescription medication?

Notes:

38. How is Pancuronium Bromide medication supposed to help me?

Notes:

39. How should I dispose of Pancuronium Bromide

prescription drugs?

Notes:

**40. How effective is this treatment?**

Notes:

41. How should I take this Pancuronium Bromide medication?

Notes:

**42. Are there support groups for people with this problem and how would I contact them?**

Notes:

**43. How soon should I come back?**

Notes:

44. How long do I need to take the Pancuronium Bromide medicine for?

Notes:

**45. How is the test done?**

Notes:


46. How is the Pancuronium Bromide medication delivered?

Notes:


47. So how do I save money on my Pancuronium Bromide prescription drugs?

Notes:


48. How should I take my Pancuronium Bromide medication?

Notes:


49. How often will I take the Pancuronium Bromide medication?

Notes:

**50. How many patients with my condition have you treated?**

Notes:

51. How will Pancuronium Bromide affect the other medications that I'm taking?

Notes:

52. How can I opt for the generic alternative Pancuronium Bromide medication that gives me the exact same results?

Notes:

53. State prescription drug price web sites, how useful are they to me as a Pancuronium Bromide consumer?

Notes:

**54. How will I hear about my test results?**

Notes:

**55. How's my weight?**

Notes:

**56. How soon do I need to have the test?**

Notes:

**57. How quickly do I have to start the treatment?**

Notes:

58. How does Pancuronium Bromide interact with other medications?

Notes:

59. How do I read the label on my Pancuronium Bromide prescription drug package?

Notes:

**60. How do I know if I have permanent hair loss due to medication?**

Notes:

61. How do I take this Pancuronium Bromide medication?

Notes:

**62. In case I need pain relief, how can I get access to medical cannabis?**

Notes:

63. How common is Pancuronium Bromide prescription drug abuse?

Notes:

**64. How can I support my bone health naturally with and without medication?**

Notes:

65. How should this Pancuronium Bromide medication be stored?

Notes:

**66. How can my mental state successfully improve using medication or therapy?**

Notes:


**67. How accurate are the results of the test?**

Notes:


68. How do I manage multiple prescription medications together with Pancuronium Bromide?

Notes:


69. How long will the effect of Pancuronium Bromide medication last?

Notes:


70. How long does the prescription drug Pancuronium Bromide stay in your system?

Notes:

71. How do you handle children on Pancuronium Bromide medication?

Notes:


72. How long should I take Pancuronium Bromide medication?

Notes:


73. How long do I have to take Pancuronium Bromide medication?

Notes:


74. How long does a Pancuronium Bromide medication remain active in your body?

Notes:


75. How can Pancuronium Bromide prescription drug abuse be recognized and stopped?

Notes:


76. How to go about it if I want to use a lower dosage

of Pancuronium Bromide?

Notes:

77. How does a person with dementia, living alone, manage her Pancuronium Bromide medication?

Notes:

**78. How will I get the test results?**

Notes:

79. How will Pancuronium Bromide affect my sleeping pattern?

Notes:

80. How do the police suspect impairment by Pancuronium Bromide prescription medication?

Notes:

# CHAPTER #7: HOW MUCH:

INTENT: How much will taking Pancuronium Bromide cost me (In money and Pancuronium Bromide's effect on quality of life.)

1. Can you take expired Pancuronium Bromide medications or not?

Notes:

2. Will Pancuronium Bromide interact with any other medicines I take - including any vitamins - herbal medicine or other complementary medicine?

Notes:

3. How much do I need to really understand about the interactions of my Pancuronium Bromide prescription drugs?

Notes:

4. What if my religion condones the use of Pancuronium Bromide medications?

Notes:

5. How much does it normally cost to get the surgery done, including all Pancuronium Bromide medications and tests (ultrasounds,x-rays,medicines, hospital stay)?

Notes:

6. How much will the plan cover for Pancuronium Bromide prescription drugs?

Notes:

7. Is _____ normal to get after only been taking the Pancuronium Bromide medication for a few days?

Notes:

8. Do I have to pay for my own Pancuronium Bromide

prescription drugs?

Notes:


**9. How much will the treatment cost?**

Notes:


10. Is there a Medicare Advantage plan provider who will cover my Pancuronium Bromide prescription drug costs during the donut hole?

Notes:


11. Are there any other precautions or warnings for this Pancuronium Bromide medication?

Notes:


12. Which Pancuronium Bromide medications are addictive?

Notes:


13. Has anyone ever used this Pancuronium Bromide medication?

Notes:



**14. Where can I make cost savings?**

Notes:



**15. How much will my Pancuronium Bromide prescription drugs cost me?**

Notes:



**16. Will Medicare be enough to cover the cost of my medical care, especially Pancuronium Bromide prescription drugs?**

Notes:



**17. Will my body get to depend upon a certain amount of my Pancuronium Bromide prescription drug, an amount that grows higher the longer I am on the drug?**

Notes:



**18. Are all drug-drug interactions limited to**

Pancuronium Bromide prescription medications?

Notes:

**19. What kinds of medications will I need to take and what if they don't work?**

Notes:

20. How do I get the Medicare Pancuronium Bromide prescription drug benefit?

Notes:

**21. How much will it cost, will the cost be covered by the PBS - my concession or Veterans Affairs card or by private health insurance?**

Notes:

22. Do pill boxes help prevent Pancuronium Bromide medication errors?

Notes:

**23. What treatments, therapies and medications**

are recommended or available for my condition?

Notes:

**24. Are medication reminders only for prescription medications?**

Notes:

**25. Should I join a Medicare Prescription Drug Plan even if I don't take many prescription drugs?**

Notes:

26. Are my Pancuronium Bromide prescription drugs FDA-approved?

Notes:

27. Should I take my Pancuronium Bromide medications at a regular time each day?

Notes:

28. Where can I obtain a list of Pancuronium Bromide prescription drugs that require prior approval?

Notes:

29. How much do the Pancuronium Bromide prescription drugs cost in this plan as compared to other plans?

Notes:

30. Regarding dosage, exactly how much of Pancuronium Bromide can I take?

Notes:

31. Can Canadian drug pharmacies mail my Pancuronium Bromide prescription drugs and medications to me?

Notes:

32. How much am I likely to spend on Pancuronium Bromide prescription drugs?

Notes:

**33. Are my prescription drugs also available in a**

**generic version?**

Notes:


**34. I am on prescription Pancuronium Bromide medication, can I still detox?**

Notes:


**35. Do I really need this treatment?**

Notes:


**36. Are there less intrusive, harmless and effective solutions instead of Pancuronium Bromide prescription drugs?**

Notes:


**37. Will I require any Pancuronium Bromide prescription drugs?**

Notes:


**38. Which Pancuronium Bromide prescription drugs can be addictive?**

Notes:



**39. Will the cost be covered by Medicare - my concession or Veterans Affairs card or by private health insurance?**

Notes:



40. Could any of the Pancuronium Bromide medications contribute to impotence?

Notes:



41. Will my gender or ethnic group be denied Pancuronium Bromide medications that work better for other groups but not for my ethnic or gender group?

Notes:



42. Could thePancuronium Bromide prescription drug I am taking now be the cause of a few extra pounds?

Notes:

43. How much Pancuronium Bromide medication can be brought through customs in case I travel?

Notes:

44. I am paid to _____ for a living, will my performance improve or decrease while using Pancuronium Bromide prescription drugs?

Notes:

45. How to get my Pancuronium Bromide medication increased?

Notes:

**46. How much will this cost me?**

Notes:

47. Which part of Medicare will cover my Pancuronium Bromide prescription drugs?

Notes:

**48. How much will the test cost?**

Notes:

49. How much should I be charged for my Pancuronium Bromide prescription medications?

Notes:

**50. Is it covered by Medicare - my concession or Veterans Affairs card or my private health insurance?**

Notes:

51. Can using too much or too little Pancuronium Bromide prescription drugs harm my health?

Notes:

**52. Should I take medication to lower my blood pressure?**

Notes:

53. Just how much do you know about the numerous types of Pancuronium Bromide medications for the

different types of my condition?

Notes:

54. What is the effect of my Pancuronium Bromide use if I smoke?

Notes:

55. How does a Pancuronium Bromide medication reminder service work?

Notes:

56. If I need a surgery and I did go ahead with the surgery, how might that affect the Pancuronium Bromide medications I take?

Notes:

**57. How much experience with this test or procedure do you have?**

Notes:

58. How do I know how much my Pancuronium

Bromide prescription medication will be?

Notes:


**59. Is it possible to lower my blood pressure without taking prescription drugs?**

Notes:


60. Do Pancuronium Bromide medications work for everybody?

Notes:


61. Will Pancuronium Bromide interfere with other prescription medications?

Notes:


62. How much is Medicare Pancuronium Bromide prescription drug coverage worth?

Notes:


63. Common side effects of Pancuronium Bromide include?

Notes:


**64. Who typically, signed up for the Medicare Prescription Drug plan, are already hitting the gap in coverage known as the doughnut hole - and what is my risk of hitting the doughnut hole?**

Notes:


**65. Can you explain my options for Medicare, Medicare/Medicaid, Disability, Supplemental Insurance, Part D Prescription Drug Plans, or Medicare Billings?**

Notes:


66. How much can I use this Pancuronium Bromide prescription drug plan?

Notes:


67. How much does Pancuronium Bromide cost?

Notes:

68. How much Pancuronium Bromide prescription medication can I order from my pharmacy at one time?

Notes:

**69. Am I am worrying too much?**

Notes:

# Index

abroad 18, 70, 79
abused 100
access 88, 110
account 3
accurate 9, 111
achieved 105
active 112
activities 81
activity 43
addiction 14-15, 28, 66, 87
addictive 72, 116, 121
adherence 27
administer 18
adults 26
Advantage 116
adverse 40
advice 1, 4
Affairs 118, 122, 124
affect 43, 55, 98, 108, 113, 125
afford 31
afforded 90
alcohol 26, 67
alleged 1
allergic 38
allergies 33, 89
allergy 92
already 3, 39, 127
always 4
Amazon 3
amount 74, 117
another 3, 36, 65
answer 3, 87
answered 4
answers 5
anymore 79
anyone 116
anything 10, 25, 41, 45, 71, 73, 93
appear 1
appetite 85
approach 47, 90

approval         119
approves         13
arising 1
arrested         80
asking 3-4, 10
asleep 65
assist    20
assisted         61
associated       16
assume           3
author 1
authors 1
available        20, 29, 35-36, 48, 58, 66, 73-74, 79, 119-120
bathing          43
because          31, 72, 78
become           1, 52
before 4, 23, 46, 58, 65, 91
BEGINNING        2, 6
benefit 1, 32, 44, 48, 118
benefits         7, 24, 76
Besides 34
better   1, 3-4, 34, 79, 94, 101, 122
between          35, 65, 82
Billings  127
biologic         65
Blokdijk 1
bought 3
branded          40
brands 65
breast  15
brewers          75
Bromide          3, 5, 7-20, 22-52, 54-67, 69-82, 84-128
brought          123
builds   3
button 3
buying 55, 76, 95
Canada           59
Canadian         120
cannabis         110
caused           1
causes 22, 33
causing          42
caution          90

certain 70, 117
change           14, 33, 46, 60
changed          49, 85
changes          16, 33
CHAPTER          2, 7, 22, 54, 69, 84, 98, 114
CHAPTERS         2, 6
charge 5
charged          124
cheaper          77
checkup          5
chemical         44
children         66, 112
choice 20, 44
chronic          63
citizens 9
claimed          1, 44
client   3
cognition        64
combine          96
combined         77, 91
common           63, 110, 126
companies        1
compare          102
compared         120
comply           18
components       39
compounds        44
concerned        60
concerns         4
concession       118, 122, 124
condition        5, 11, 29-30, 33, 35, 43, 51, 59, 63, 70, 75, 82, 92-93, 97-99, 101, 103, 105, 108, 119, 125
conditions       9, 79
condones         115
confidence       9
consider         76
considered       80
construed        1
consumer         108
consumers        1
contact          11, 79, 106
contained        1
container        80

| | |
|---|---|
| contains | 4 |
| Contents | 2 |
| continual | 3 |
| continue | 19 |
| contribute | 122 |
| convey | 1 |
| co-pays | 87 |
| Copyright | 1 |
| correct | 17 |
| counseling | 25 |
| counter | 35, 58, 67, 93 |
| course | 33 |
| coverage | 10, 14, 41, 50, 57, 64, 76, 93, 103-104, 126-127 |
| covered | 18, 27, 65, 70, 97, 118, 122, 124 |
| creams | 19 |
| create | 3, 18 |
| current | 33, 54, 56, 59, 70, 79, 89, 96, 103 |
| currently | 47, 93 |
| Customer | 3 |
| customs | 123 |
| damage | 1 |
| dangerous | 52, 95, 97 |
| Database | 11 |
| decrease | 123 |
| deductible | 85 |
| delivered | 107 |
| dementia | 113 |
| denied | 122 |
| depend | 117 |
| dependent | 45 |
| depending | 67 |
| depends | 3 |
| depression | 66 |
| described | 1 |
| detected | 98 |
| determine | 44 |
| diagnose | 20 |
| difference | 35 |
| different | 24, 99, 125 |
| difficult | 27 |
| difficulty | 24 |
| directions | 27 |
| directly | 1 |

Disability      127
discard 19
disclaim        1
Disclaimer      1
discuss 5
disease         35
dispose         26, 50, 102-103, 105
doctor 3-4, 13, 23, 41, 81
doctors         4, 70
dosage          112, 120
dosages         1, 32
doughnut        127
drinking        8
drinks  24, 81
drowsiness      28
drug-drug       117
during  48, 61, 71, 80, 116
easiest 50
eating 8
editorial       1
effect  11, 17, 26, 28, 31, 33, 42, 57, 80, 111, 114, 125
effective       4, 57, 65, 76, 87, 106, 121
effects 16, 22, 28, 30, 34, 40, 44-45, 49-52, 57-59, 62, 64, 72, 77, 93, 95, 126
effort  4
either  69
electronic      1
eligible 10
emergency       79
employees       64
employer        36, 56, 64
enough          60, 117
entity  1
enzymes         14, 18
equipment       27
errors  28, 118
especially      3, 75, 117
ethnic  122
evaluate        97
everybody       126
Everyone        3
everything      4
everywhere      80

evidence 38, 61
exactly 13, 45, 91, 120
examples 3
excessive 76
exercise 39, 48
expect 22-23, 28, 40, 42, 95
expensive 57
experience 47, 50, 125
expiration 52
expire 82
expired 114
explain 65, 86, 127
explore 55
family 86
fashion 1
faster 65
feedback 2-3
females 22, 57
filled 57, 67
financial 73
finding 13
flow-on 66
follow 3, 16
following 8
forever 61
forget 7, 47
formulary 54
fulfil 47
function 62
further 20
gender 122
generic 11-12, 26, 33, 58, 63, 65-66, 78, 82, 102, 108, 121
generics 20
getting 3, 5, 57, 62, 75, 93, 96
giving 89
Googled 9
graduate 77
grapefruit 55, 90
groups 106, 122
habits 8, 85
handle 66, 112
happen 39, 42, 48, 88
happens 31, 37, 41, 46, 54, 59

harmed 12
harmful 52
harmless 121
having 3, 19, 24, 81, 100
healing 46
health 1, 3-5, 40, 42, 60, 71, 79, 97, 110, 118, 122, 124
healthy 35
helping 60
herbal 56, 70, 114
herein 1
higher 117
highlight 4
history 86, 89
hitting 127
hospital 115
identified 1
illegal 9
impairment 113
important 3-5, 22, 37, 91
impotence 122
improve 3, 70, 93, 111, 123
improves 75
include 126
included 44
including 89, 114-115
increased 123
indirectly 1
individual 96
informed 1
instead 91, 121
instructed 69
insurance 27, 90, 118, 122, 124, 127
intended 1
INTENT 7, 22, 54, 69, 84, 98, 114
intention 1
interact 15, 51, 73, 75, 109, 114
interfere 91, 126
internet 58
intrusive 121
invaluable 2-3
involve 23
involved 81
irritable 55

issues   47
itself   1
latest   50
legally   9, 59
liability   1
lifestyle 33
likely   15, 79, 98, 120
limited 4, 54, 117
listed   1
little   36, 49, 124
living   61, 113, 123
locally   57
longer 31, 73, 117
long-term   11
making   49
manage   94, 101-102, 111, 113
management 11, 39
market 52
matter 9, 86
matters   1
mechanical   1
Medicaid   127
medical   1, 4-5, 14, 59, 77, 86-87, 89, 92, 110, 117
Medicare   8, 10, 20, 41, 103, 116-119, 122-124, 126-127
medicate   84
medication   7, 9-18, 20, 23, 25-27, 29-37, 39-40, 42-45, 47-52, 56-60, 63, 65-67, 69-71, 73-82, 84-88, 90-95, 97-101, 104-113, 115-116, 118-119, 121, 123-126, 128
medicinal   24
medicine   5, 20, 61, 78, 85, 106, 114
medicines   33, 69, 114-115
meditation   51
members   4
mental 18, 111
mention   1
messed   86
methods   105
Monitoring   11
monitors   88
mud-bath   11
multiple   27, 111
natural 19, 38, 57, 67, 69, 76, 81, 88, 97
naturally   110

nature 26, 55
nausea 17, 80
necessary 15
negative 25, 58
negatively 98
neither 1
neuritis 64
normal 7, 70, 115
normally 115
Notice 1
number 129
numerous 4, 124
nursing 34
obtain 50, 90, 119
offers 4
Off-label 10
ointments 19, 35
ongoing 11
online 3, 8-9, 51, 96
opinion 63
opioid 55
opionion 54
optimum 55
options 10, 24, 41, 43, 45, 56, 127
others 55, 94, 96
otherwise 1
outcome 23, 39
outside 80
overdose 31
overseas 47
package 109
parents 26
particular 91
partner 66
patient 14, 101
patients 61, 69, 108
pattern 113
paying 24
people 1, 70, 106
percent 25
perform 100
period 49
permanent 57, 109

permission 1
person 1, 18, 113
personal 89
pharmacies 120
pharmacy 8, 128
physician 1
Please 65
pocket 80
police 113
policies 96
popular 87
positive 32, 61, 89
possible 36, 57, 64, 126
potent 19
potential 66
pounds 122
precaution 1
precise 1
Precisely 92
pregnancy 48, 61
pregnant 20, 75
prepare 4
prepared 5
prescribe 1, 59, 70, 82
prescribed 26, 31, 56, 84, 91-92
prescribes 3
pressing 4
pressure 62, 124, 126
prevent 7, 26, 30, 35, 71, 118
prices 72, 89
primary 91
private 118, 122, 124
proactive 3
probable 98
problem 5, 20, 91, 98, 106
problems 8, 15, 18, 60, 100
procedure 42, 58-59, 125
procedures 3, 43
process 3
produce 52
product 1, 3
products 1, 24, 76
programs 87

proper 33, 94
properly 102
provider 116
providers 3, 5
provides 5, 76
providing 3
publisher 1
purchase 3, 13, 59
purchased 3
qualified 11, 96
quality 3, 102, 114
question 2-3, 6, 41
questions 3-5, 27
quickly 109
reaction 38
readily 79
really 46, 60, 74, 84, 92, 114, 121
reason 5, 91
reasons 30, 32, 92
receive 10-11, 61
receiving 25
recently 3
recognized 112
recommend 24, 27, 29, 48, 95
recording 1
Records 16
recurring 30
reduce 100, 104
references 129
refuse 56
regarding 1, 8, 120
regimen 18
regular 23-24, 119
regularly 90
related 28
relation 43, 48
relevant 3
relief 36, 49, 86, 110
religion 115
remain 112
remedies 35, 52, 55, 81, 88
remedy 43
remember 37

remind 76
reminder 125
reminders 20, 88, 119
replace 1
reproduced 1
requested 1
requests 81
require 1, 65, 93, 96, 119, 121
required 46
research 89
reserved 1
resources 36
respect 1
response 28
result 25, 32
results 3, 40, 72, 75, 89, 100, 108, 111, 113
review 3, 20
reviews 3
revisit 8
rights 1
ringing 24
rushed 4
safely 19, 81, 102
safest 26, 50
safety 3, 88
savings 117
school 71, 77, 90
scientists 44
second 54, 63
sellers 1
seniors 74
serious 22, 103
service 3, 125
services 1, 27
sexual 28
sharing 9
should 1, 3-4, 7, 10, 12, 16, 20, 23-24, 27, 31, 33, 39, 41-43, 46, 50-51, 57-58, 60-63, 67, 69, 71, 74-76, 78-82, 84, 86, 96, 99, 105-107, 110, 112, 119, 124
shrink 7
signed 127
simple 4
simpler 10

simply 3
situation 4, 25
sleeping 113
smoking 8
solution 57
solutions 121
someone 14, 100
soreness 43
sources 25, 29, 51
specialist 11, 89
specific 3
stated 80
stocked 105
stolen 35
stopped 16, 112
stored 110
stranded 70
strength 94
subject 3
submitted 14
substance 66
substances 89
suddenly 88
suffer 63
suffering 87
suggest 28
supplement 1
supplies 61
support 81, 106, 110
supposed 101, 105
surgeries 100
surgery 5, 9, 29, 78-79, 115, 125
surgical 43
suspect 113
switching 58, 65
symptoms 9, 28, 42, 70, 74, 84, 91, 99
system 111
taking 8, 15-19, 22, 29, 31, 33, 36-37, 43, 46-47, 49, 55-56, 62-64, 69, 75-76, 80-82, 88, 90-91, 97-98, 108, 114-115, 122, 126
Talking 3
testing 20
themselves 74
therapies 29, 70, 118

therapy         60, 78, 111
things   4
thoughts        30
through         123
throughout      1, 95
together        40, 64, 78, 81, 111
toxins   92
trademark       1
trademarks      1
trained 1
travel   97, 123
travelling      47
treated         108
treating        91
treatment       7, 18, 24-25, 33, 38, 41, 46, 49, 87, 99, 101, 106, 109, 116, 121
treatments      87, 118
trying   36
typically       8, 127
unable 18, 88
underlying      92
understand      27, 114
unhappy         40
unused 50
unwanted        26, 45
unwelcome       52
useful   51, 108
validating      17
various 52, 89
varying 34
version 63, 78, 121, 129
Veterans        118, 122, 124
visits    13
vitamin 56
vitamins        31, 43, 46, 73, 114
vomiting        80
waiting 49
warnings        22, 37, 116
warranty        1
weight 43, 77, 109
Whatever        5
whether         44
wholesome       11

willing  59
without 1, 14, 19, 39, 45, 90, 93, 95, 98, 101, 105, 110, 126
working     13, 48, 59, 71, 79, 82
worried     96
worrying    128
worsening   30
writing 3
written 1
x-rays   115
yeasts  75
yourself    4, 34, 46

Made in the USA
Monee, IL
26 July 2021